How to Be a Good Home Nurse

Tips on your family's health

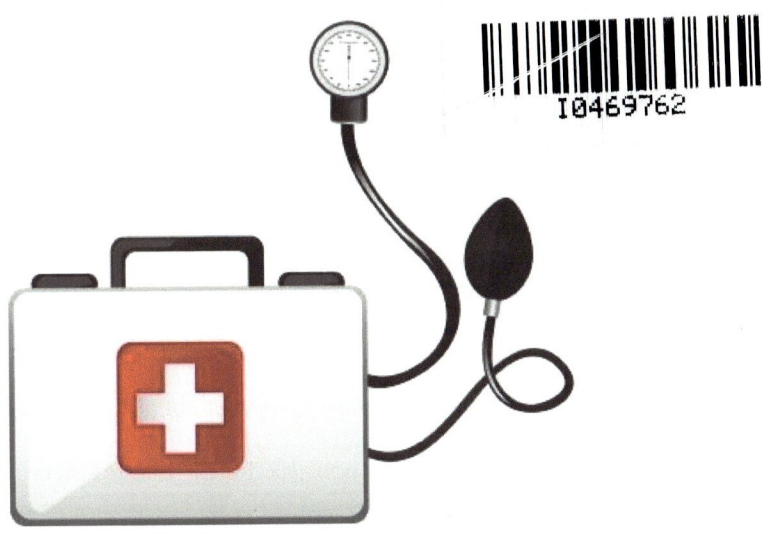

Dueep Jyot Singh

Natural Remedy Series

Mendon Cottage Books

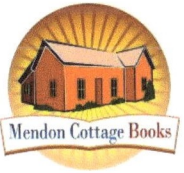

JD-Biz Publishing

Our books are available at

1. Amazon.com
2. Barnes and Noble
3. Itunes
4. Kobo
5. Smashwords
6. Google Play Books

Table of Contents

Introduction

Each of us is growing older with every passing moment, and most of us subconsciously have a nagging worry about who is going to take care of us, when we get old or when we are sick. Women, far more than men dread the idea of growing old. That is because they subconsciously have the fear that there will be nobody to take care of them, then they grow comparatively old and helpless. The first adjustment to this idea comes in middle age, with its foreshadowing of old age. This is when middle-aged people begin to think about the next stage of life.

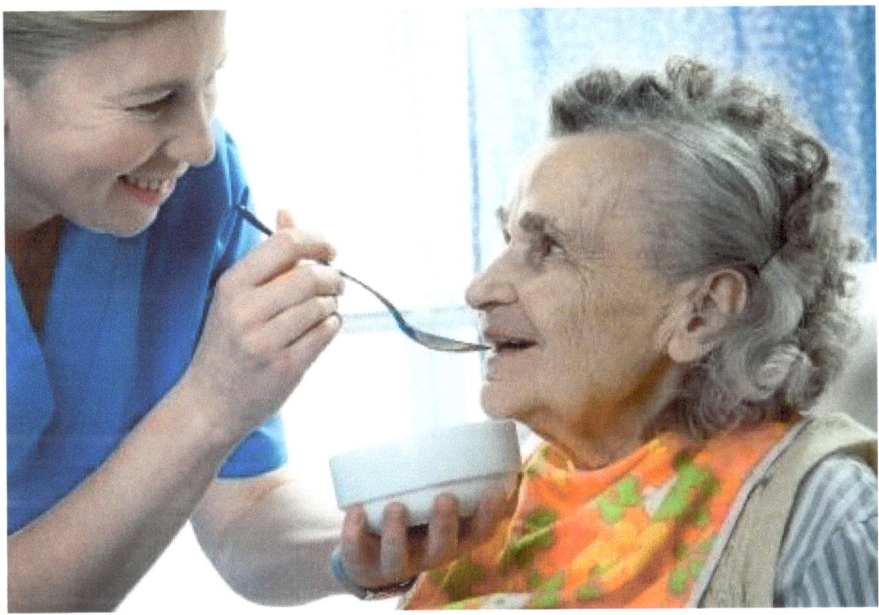

If a woman has devoted her life to being the center of her family, she may look ahead fearfully to the days to come, when her children will be adults and will have flown the nest. If she has a happy married life, she knows that she has her partner, who is going to grow old with her. But unfortunately sometimes it just happens that homes break up and many people find themselves approaching middle age, and future old age, in loneliness. That is when they begin to take good care of their finances so that they have enough of money, which they can utilize when they are old.

Among all the impermanent and threatening shadows of the days to come, a woman may have before her the example of some cantankerous old lady who has become an unloved, and unwelcome burden to her children demanding and less attention from some already hard-pressed daughter-in-law or daughter.

And this condition worsens, if that person is ill. In the East, where the idea of sending parents to an old-age home, is still something of which one thinks of with loathing and abhorrence, nursing of the eldest generation is done at home. Affluent families keep home nurses who are professional. Other not so affluent families take care of the elders, not because it is their duty, but because it is part of the Eastern and Oriental social fabric, coming down the ages.

However, this idea is slowly being eroded in many cities, because the children are more bothered about making money, instead of giving proper care to their elders. The elders also try their best to keep away from under the children's feet and make sure that they are financially secure. The day of the joint family is slowly and steadily disappearing, when the younger generations used to take care of the older generations.

It is often said by Easterners, that in many countries in the West, they have lost the sense of filial duty, which still exists in so many Latin and Eastern countries. This is where old people are respected and taken into their children's homes. Westerners are often accused of heartlessness, because so often they send their parents away to live the rest of their lives in an old peoples home. This may be right, but one cannot generalize.

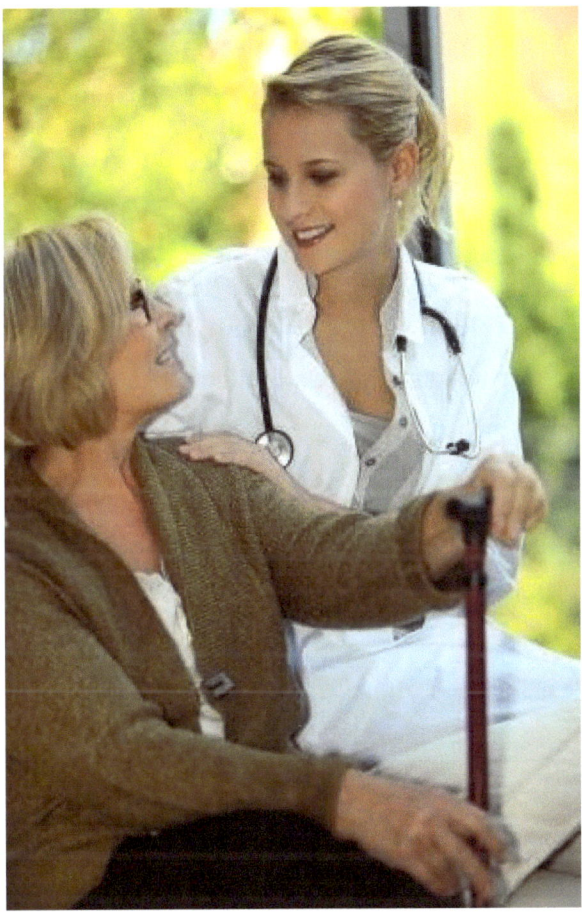

Nursing Homes are getting to be more and more common in the West

Nevertheless, there are so many families still in the West, where the children take care of their parents and I know of many of them. That is why I say that idea of carelessness and apathy and selfishness is not a true statement .

However, sometimes in today's hectic environment, heavy burdens are already placed on young shoulders. The younger generation, often finds it necessary to go out to work as well as looking after the members of the family – both the young and old – and however much the old one is loved, one more straw is often all that it takes to break the camel's back.

That is why they prefer that the responsibility of full-time care of the older generation is so often left in the hands of professional old peoples homes. Although we keep on hearing about scandals of inadequately managed homes where old people are badly treated, just like as they were treated in Charles Dickens age and times, there are still many homes where the residents are happy in the care of kind and loving staff.

In some cases where an old person is suffering from an infirmity or illness which demands constant nursing, there is no possible solution other than full-time care which a qualified staff can give and a harassed family cannot.

Yet one knows that wherever old people reside, they are themselves the authors of the care and love which they receive. It is to some extent up to them whether they are visited only out of a sense of duty or because those who come to see them love visiting and being with them. It is their choice whether they make themselves a burden or a bonus to their families.

A lovable old person is a loving old person who wants to be with, or as close as possible to, loved ones, yet is determined never to become a burden or make further demands on the limited resources and limited time of those loved ones. All this is done not just through pride, or wanting to stand on one's own feet, but out of love and concern for them.

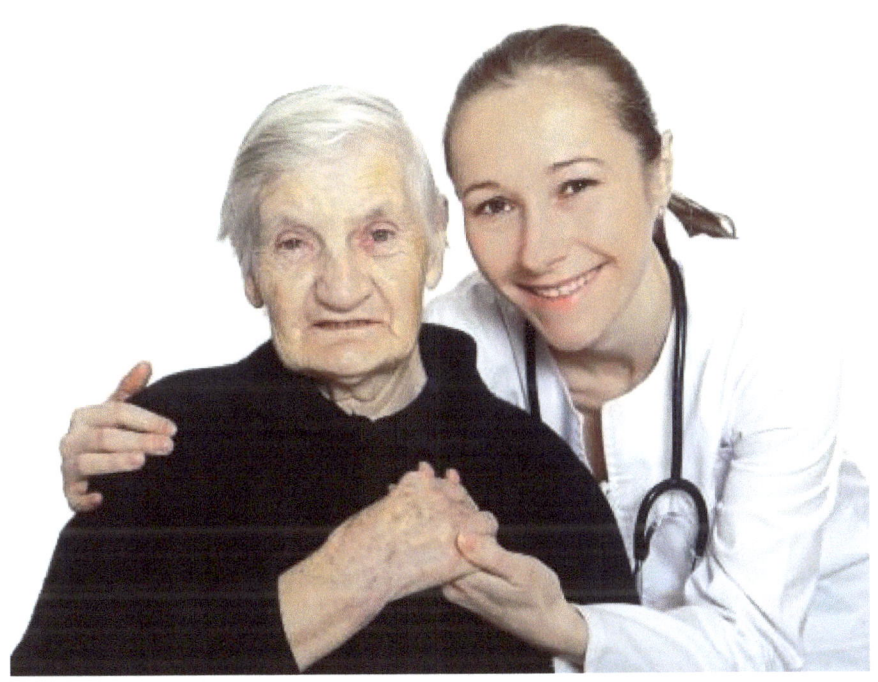

Life is worth living! With people who care around you.

There was a time when the elders were the autocrats of the family. That is why the younger generation considered it their duty to respond to every call, notwithstanding the fact that some of the elder generation were demanding, cantankerous, tyrannical and difficult. They were also capable of ordering their children to drop everything in order to help them on any problem, however trivial. And the children had to do that, just because that older generation had the purse strings firmly grasped in their hands.

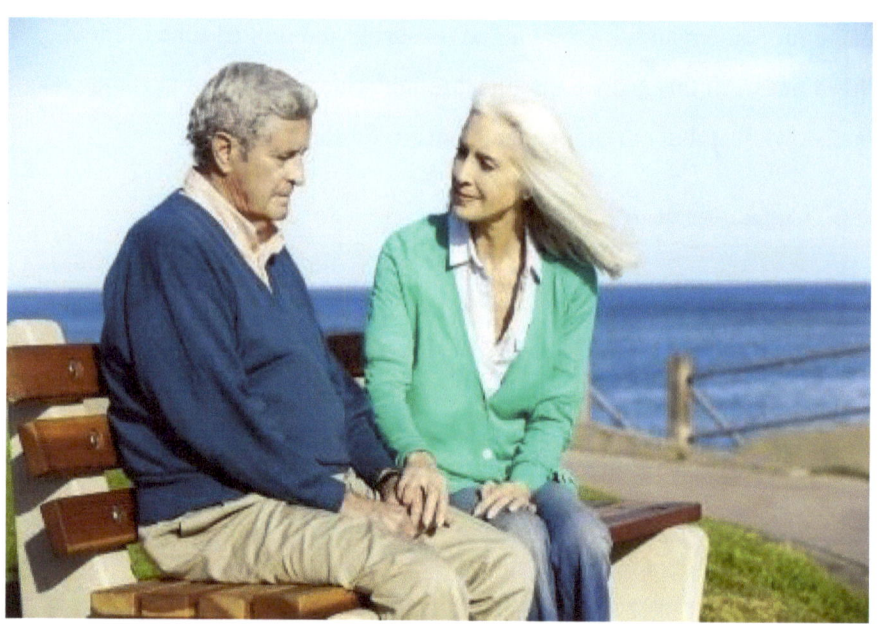

The coming sunset of our years is the time when we need care and support.

But that is not so nowadays. Children are independent, and raise their own families in their own nuclear world. They are not dependent on their parents for financial help. And that is why the idea of a duty to a parent is slowly being forgotten, notwithstanding the social traditions, and familial upbringing.

So when somebody talks about old people, and their nursing and care, many people say – well, we will just put them in the hospital when such a situation occurs, because we can afford to do so. Or we shall employ a full-time nurse at home.

But many times, that is not possible. Also, many times the hospital personnel tell the family – "we have done all we can, now it is time for home nursing. So, take the patient home." I have seen that being done many times in large and reputed hospitals, where they are more bothered about getting beds free for more patients.

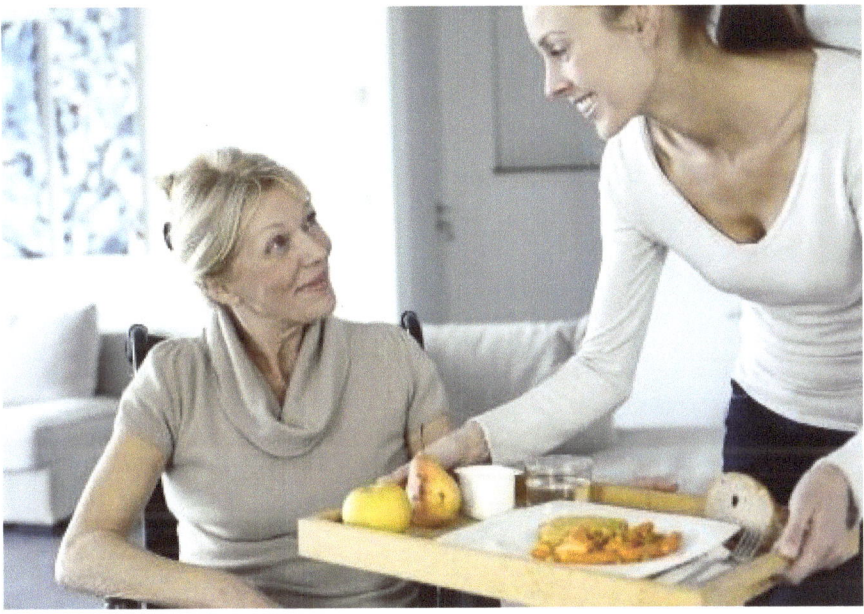

On the other hand, hospitals are sometimes dumping grounds for patients, who are getting to be burdens for people who do not want to take on the responsibility of caring for the old and elderly. And then it depends on how dedicated a doctor is and how much he cares about the patient, before he signs the papers of release sending the patient back home.

I am saying this, because I have seen that happening, in 1995, when I was working as a hospital administrator for my cousin's cardio- Gynae hospital. This episode is rather tragic, because things like this happen in hospitals all over the world.

One evening, a patient about 85 years old, was admitted by his daughter-in-law. She had to go on a holiday with her "friend" for a couple of days, and as her husband was away on a business trip abroad, it was the responsibility of the doctor and the nurses to take care of her father-in-law.

My sister-in-law told me to admit him, even though my cousin brother, the cardiologist, had checked him up and said that there was nothing wrong with him. In this manner, at least, he would get 3 to 5 days of rest and good food in a caring atmosphere.

So the lady went away. But unfortunately for her, the father died the next day. And even worse, the husband came back unexpectedly and came straight to the hospital. He had heard from his neighbors that his father had been admitted in our hospital, and where was his wife?

I was a completely tactless and naive brute in those days. And so innocently, I told him that he had been admitted here, two nights ago because his wife had to go on a holiday with some of her friends and she was not picking up the phone. It was good that he was here, because he could take charge of his father.

He listened open mouthed and shocked. He was under the impression that his wife was taking good care of his father. Not so, said a nurse. Every time he went on tour, she went on a holiday and dumped her father in law here.

You could say that she was also tactless and brutal! But then, we are taught to be that when we have to do some straight talking to people who shirk their responsibilities or put their own responsibilities on the shoulders of somebody else who could not care less.

And things like that do not happen in real life, but this happened. The 17,000 in one chance.

He was still sitting in my office, when the wife walked in. She had come to take her father-in-law back.

I went to meet her in the reception room, and told her about his sad demise.

Dead, no, no, that cannot be. Now, what would she say to her husband?

Up she picked a chair, and smash went a window of the reception room.

And then she began berating my cousin by saying that he was supposed to be an experienced and well-known cardiologist. Her "dear father" was perfectly well when she had left him in the hospital, so how did he die? How could Dr. Sahib let him die?

The answer was, "If he was perfectly well, why did you think he needed to be brought here to the hospital?" said my cousin, reasonably.

"Ummmm, well, he was feeling some discomfort so I decided that he should be brought here to the hospital. He was your responsibility, then. You have taken good care of him before. Besides, I did not want to leave him alone at home. I am sure he was very serious, and that is why he died. Yes, that is it, and you should have taken care of him. You should have. You should have." All the while, weeping gustily and disturbing the rest of other patients.

"If you thought that he was feeling some discomfort or if you were sure that he was really "serious," was it really necessary for you to go running off to your party? Could not you just sit here by his side, if he was in such a worry making state? You could have yelled for us, if you felt he was going into cardiac arrest. We would have saved him. "

I was standing there and I could not resist adding my own mite with this hysterical vixen making such a noise in our hospital.

My cousin shushed me because I was being typically and thoroughly insensitive, but this woman had been creating and accusing my cousin of neglect and I had lost patience with her. She hoped that this would protect her from the wrath of her husband, to whom this story would be conveyed with plenty of spice, mustard and pepper. And her husband was listening to each and every word we spoke…

He then came out of my office and saw the windowpane that she had broken to show everybody how much she cared for her father-in-law, who had died due to the neglect of a doctor. And then he looked at her…

The rest of the story need not to be told but can be understood.

Now this woman belonged to a very affluent family. She could have afforded a full-time nurse. So could her husband. But she wanted to show everybody that she took such good care of her father-in-law. And her husband thought that. The old man did not complain, because he knew that if he did so, he would be treated even worse, when his son went away again as he did so often. That is why she had got into the habit of admitting him into the hospital, while she went out to celebrate with her friend. And the old man never opened his mouth, out of fear.

Now, if she had been in the West, she would have immediately sued my cousin for malpractice. And she would have won. And a doctor, however experienced, he was, would have no say in the matter. Because he had failed in his Oath of Hippocrates that of keeping the patient alive. He had supposedly neglected an old person who had died in the hospital. So he was to blame.

But as that happened in the East, and everybody knew about that woman and her family and her "friend" and her way of treating her husband's widower father, the sympathy was with my cousin. In addition, because the husband was there, his reaction was, "Why did you not tell me that she did this regularly to my father." My cousin gave him a "Grow up and do not be such a dimwit, it is time you walk up to your own behavior and actions." Look.

It was not a doctor's responsibility to interfere in somebody else's family life. His job was to take care of his patients.

This was something I had never come across before. And when I asked my sister-in-law if this was an isolated case, she said, seriously and cynically, "hey this happens all the time here. This is real life."

So this is what happens often with people who are sick. Nobody seems to care about them. And then those irresponsible people go into the blame game to assuage their feelings of guilt or out of sheer fear of social censure.

So let us come back to more pleasant things, and tips and techniques on dedicated, and caring home nursing done not only to the elders, but also to any sick member in our family, be he a child or an adult.

It is surprising that women are the first people to defend the slightest insinuation that they are not aware of their own family's health. Yet we often find that most women do not recognize warning health signals when serious problems occur in the family. It is only natural that many of us can and do make mistakes, some which are too obvious to be pointed out. Yet we continue to, sadly, neglect the common precautions taken to avoid such events.

Failure to Follow a Doctor's Instructions

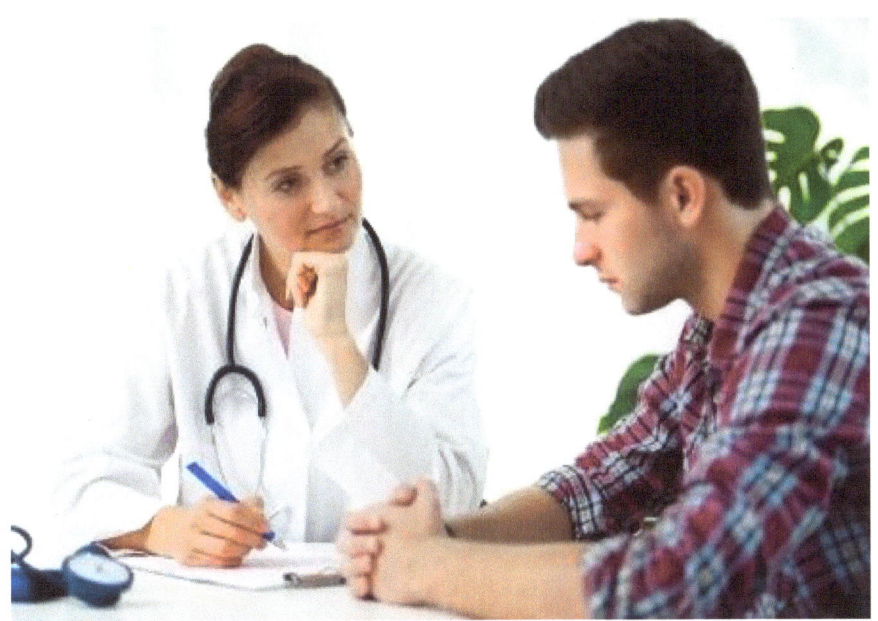

Never ignore your doctor's advice or recommendations. It is your responsibility to take care of your and your family's health.

You may go to the best doctor or hospital with the best medical treatment available, but if you do not follow the instructions in the matters of rest, diet and other precautions, which will help the patient recover faster, it will be of no use at all.

For this, it is necessary that notes should be taken about all the medical instructions, which need to be followed strictly. Never ignore your doctor's orders because he has more experience than you would ever have. Make sure that they are followed in that particular order.

Rest and Quiet for Your Patient

People do not understand that this is necessary even for minor ailments and much better than dosing your patient with chemical-based drugs. Sleep is the best restorer and healer. That is why healers in ancient times give most of their patients sleeping droughts made about herbs. Unfortunately, this practice was misused in 18th and 19th century England, where patients were put to sleep with laudanum by housewives, because that was the way in which they could get peace and quiet. Doctors also prescribed laudanum, when patients were in pain.

 Laudanum was based on opium, and opium is addictive. Such patients then became addicted to opium and could not sleep even when they were well, without a dose of laudanum.

So make sure that your patient gets plenty of natural sleep, without giving him sleeping tablets. Failure to follow this golden rule will immediately have a diverse effect upon their health. The fever may not go away completely, and you may see a relapse after a few days.

You can make your doctor's life easier by following his instructions diligently. Some people think it unwise to rest, because they are under the impression that being "up and about" helps in the recovery time better. In fact, this belief has its basis on fact. In the Indian Army, any soldier suffering from fever is immediately given treatment in the hospital and then told, "all right then, soldier, up and about. No malingering. Out, out!" So unless he is at death's door, he is not encouraged to keep resting in a bed. That is going to weaken his body more. Nine times out of 10, he gets healed naturally. Never seen a 10th time in my experience!

The idea is that the more he exercises and does physical work, the more his body gets used to the fact, that it is getting well, and there is absolutely nothing wrong with it. This is a good way of autosuggestion, which has been practiced through the ages.

This is not a new concept in India or in the East, for that matter. The Spartans practiced this also millenniums ago. It was a matter of pride to show no weakness, so even when they were suffering from wounds and from fever, they did their duty till they dropped. Luckily, we are not in the age of Spartans and continuous war. We can afford to rest. But resting for every little ailment, and coddling ourselves, just because we have this tiny sniffle and dosing ourselves with medicines, just because they are easily available does not give our body a chance to heal its self naturally.

Take Your Prescribed Medicine Regularly

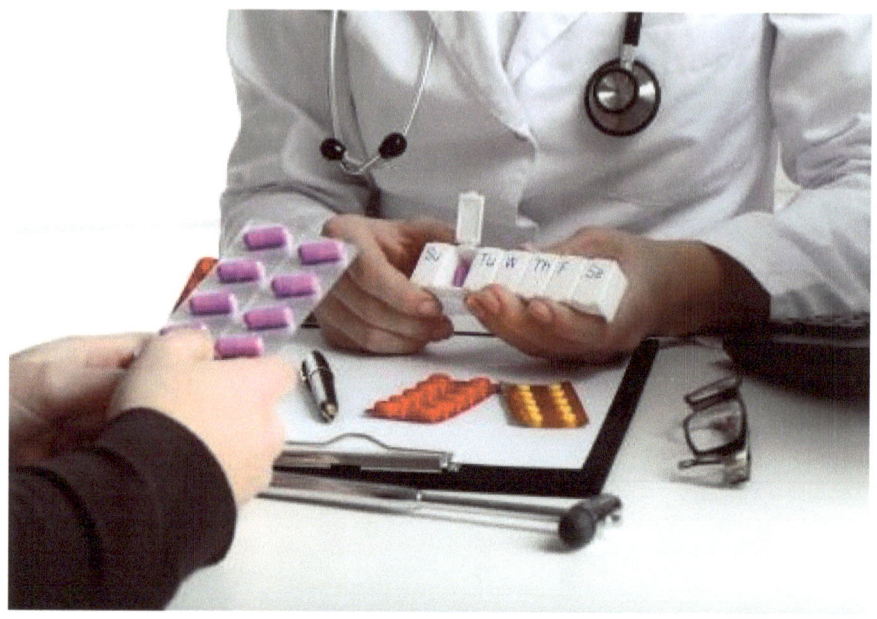

Do not stop this prescribed course midway.

Many of us have a tendency to start a course of medication and then stop it halfway as soon as we feel a bit better. It is extremely necessary that we continue the medication for the time specified by the doctor, even if the symptoms disappear before this time.

Remember that your doctor knows best. He has a good reason for specifying the dosage as well as the length of time for the medication.

A viral infection may appear again if you stop taking your medication in the middle of its prescribed course. It is necessary to regain your health completely by taking your medicine as prescribed, regularly and for the full course.

Seeking Medical Help Too Late

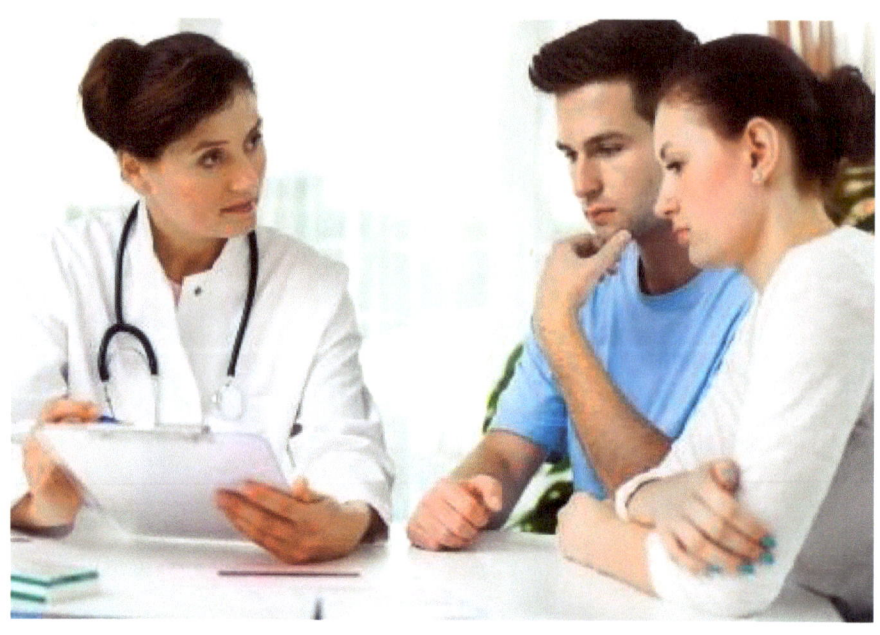

See a doctor, if you are worried about some persistent symptom.

Of course there are many among us who run to our doctor for every little cut and scratch. On the other hand, there are many of us who would not be seen dead in the hospital until absolutely necessary. And if a serious problem arises, the latter group ignores the symptoms and unfortunately that is going to have disastrous results. That is because they do not want to go to a doctor. That means that niggling pain in their stomach is possibly due to indigestion/constipation/an over fertile imagination.

You can pretend to be in the best of health, by neglecting symptoms, but being a stoic martyr and suffering in silence, just because you have been brought up that way, and you are keeping silent through a matter of pride, helps nobody, and only harms you in the long run. Being such stoic martyrs millenniums ago, was possibly fashionable and in keeping with the social traditions, conduct, comportment and beliefs of those times, but when you have medical access, which can help in treating you, why do not you take advantage of it.

When to See a Doctor

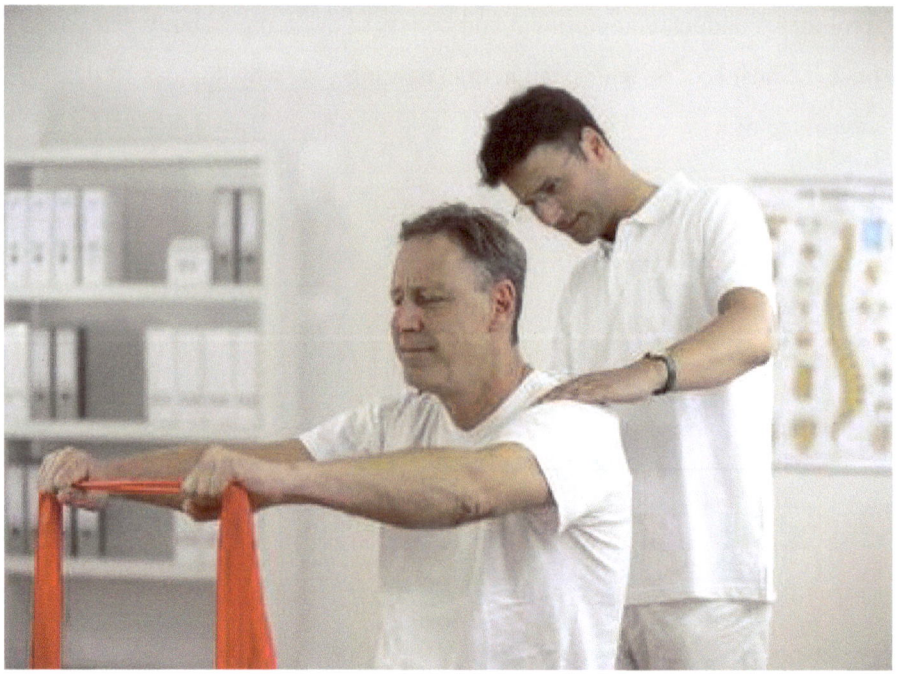

Regular checkups are good for your health.

Do not hesitate to see your doctor if the following symptoms persist –

If a high-temperature lingers for more than 24 hours, do not resort to Paracetamol or any other analgesic and hope the fever will go away. Consult your doctor immediately if your fever is more than 102°. Though I have known people going to their offices when they are suffering from fevers up to 103°, out of a matter of pride or because they are under the impression that their office is going to collapse if they are not around to manage it.

These people are not only a nuisance to their colleagues, because they could possibly be suffering from an infectious disease, but also they are harming themselves.

Instead of taking proper rest and medical advice, they are showing the world that they are doing something really praiseworthy. I do not think so. Be sensible.

If little babies are sick, take absolutely no chances, and talk to your doctor immediately.

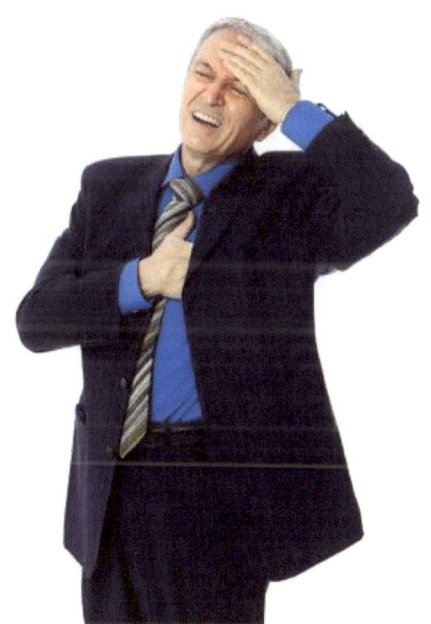

If there are sharp pains in your chest and abdomen, or a sudden, intense and painful headache, call your doctor immediately.

It is much better being told that you suffer from a tension headache or possible constipation, then find out that you had a silent heart attack. But many of us think that the doctor is going to get annoyed, because we troubled him with those trivial symptoms. If you are not in the habit of running to him, with every little symptom, he is definitely not going to be annoyed. He is going to be happy that you were careful enough about your health and contacted him.

If the symptoms persist for more than 3 to 5 days, or appear after every few days, you need to go and see your doctor again. He is going to diagnose some more tests.

It is always a mistake to hide your symptoms from your doctor, hoping they will disappear. Many a time, serious diseases have gone out of control, thanks to the reticence on the part of the patients. This normally happens when female patients are too shy to talk about their personal symptoms with their doctors, especially in the East. Just because they have not been brought up to do so. This sort of shy modesty has no place in the scheme of things, when your health is at stake.

I saw that happening, many times when my very patient gynecologist sister-in-law had to prise out the symptoms from blushing rustics, who just nodded away shyly while looking at the ground. According to them, having a disease in those "personal places" was shameful. Let the doctor Sahib do the talking.

This sort of mental outlook has no place in the 21st century in the East or in the West. But it is changing slowly, with the dissemination of knowledge and changing of mental outlooks.

An early consultation can make all the difference between life and death, treatment and despair.

For the following symptoms, go to your doctor immediately –

- Difficulty in swallowing or continued constipation.
- A bleeding wound which does not heal quite completely.
- A persistent wet cough which has been troubling you for more than 2 to 3 weeks. This may be because of a chest infection, which can be potentially dangerous.
- An unusual discharge or bleeding in any part of the body.
- A lump in any part of the body. This is going to be a soft or a hard mass of tissue.

  These are just some of the symptoms, which can be symptomatic of some other serious disease.

Overuse or misuse of Medications

This normally comes under the heading of self-medication. Look around. There are so many self-proclaimed medical practitioners, perhaps in your family also who have a quick remedy for every ailment. Some of them may be time tested, and ancient herbal recipes and they work. But others may just be quack remedies being told to you, by somebody, just because somebody else experimented with those remedies and recovered.

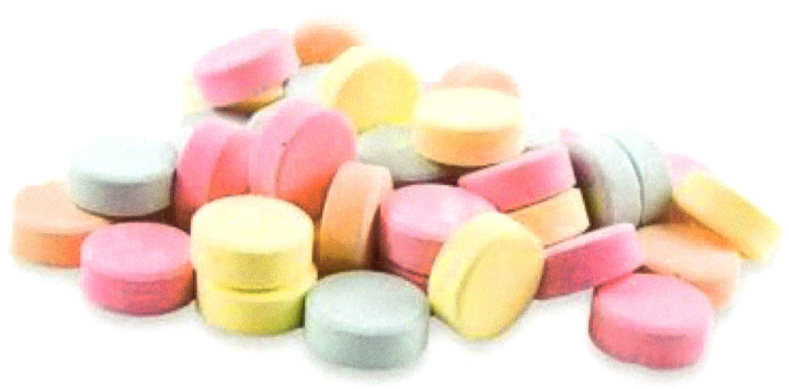

Are you a chronic pill popper?

What is sauce for the goose is definitely not always sauce for the gander. And similar symptoms do not always mean that the other person is suffering from the same disease or health problem. Besides that, you have a different biophysiological, genetic and chemical makeup from the people all around you.

Also be careful about that prevalent idea that taking more medicine than what has been prescribed will have more beneficial effects. This is dangerous and foolish.

Do not try your own remedies and nostrums if you are suffering from high fever or potentially dangerous diseases. It is very important to consult your doctor if even minor symptoms persist for more than a week.

Laxatives

The most common and misused non-prescriptive medicines are laxatives. Older people try to change their bowel habits, which are natural, and which in some people may be once every two or three days, according to the amount of green vegetables and fruits, rough fibers and grain products ingested.

Some people are under the impression that it is necessary for them to have a bowel movement every day. Because the elders said so. That is only going to happen if you have eaten enough, the previous day, to make wastes to be eliminated. And if you are not drinking enough of water, you are going to suffer from constipation. You cannot have a bowel movement the very next day, if you are subsisting on a couple of pieces of bread, cheese, some potato chips and cups of coffee for the past 24 hours. Instead, you are going to be suffering from constipation.

So if the quantity of food taken is less, your bowel movements are going to be less regular. And so you decide to take a laxative. Remember, over eating of laxatives can lead to bad health.

If you have eaten, more meat and chicken products and less of greens, you are not going to have proper bowel movement at the given time, the next day because protein products take more time to digest. But you are worried. There is something wrong with your system. You take a laxative and get rid of the half-digested food. Soon you get used to doing that and your natural bowel movement system gets disturbed.

Natural Vitamins and Chemical Supplements

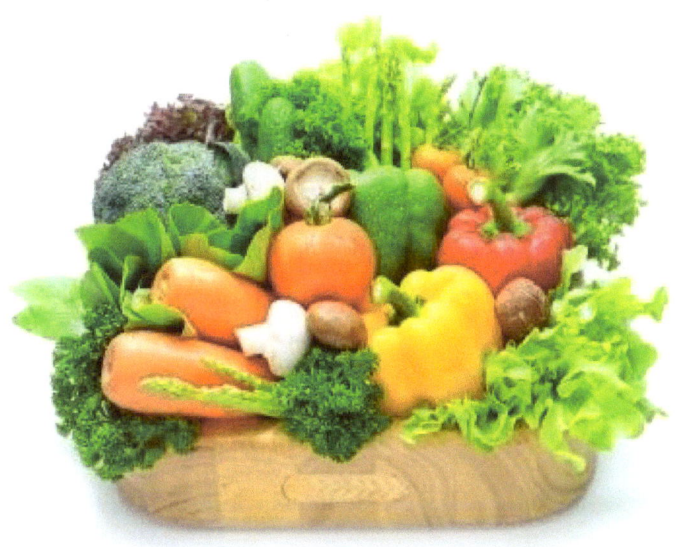

The best natural vitamins are what you get from a healthy natural diet

There is also a tendency to supplement the nutrients and vitamins in your natural food by taking extracts and pills. In fact, I know of many people, who subsist on supplements giving them vitamins instead of eating a proper natural ingredient diet. That is because they are too busy and when their body tells them that it is feeling a deficiency of some particular minerals, nutrients, and vitamins, which are necessary to keep it functioning properly, they pop a pill. Or they try out some expensive supplement endorsed by a Star.

Remember that this is going to lead to an excess of vitamins in your body, which is possibly going to cause a problem. After all, even vitamins have a definite toxic limit especially vitamin A and vitamin D.

A well-balanced diet is enough to provide all the vitamins and minerals needed by a growing body, unless prescribed by a doctor, do not take extra pills and tonics sold over the counter. Sometimes older people need some vitamins and minerals to keep in good health, but youngsters do not generally need them if they are eating a well-balanced and proper healthy nutritious diet.

Medical Records

Always keep medical records for all your family members. This is going to help in cases of emergency. This should include all records of illnesses, immunization shots and vaccines, allergy, and other relevant medical information about all the members of your family.

This is very helpful because I know of someone who suffers from an allergy to sulfa and penicillin drugs. And he found it out, when he was injected with a sulfa antibiotic in a hospital, and his body immediately went into allergic mode by swelling up. The doctors immediately gave him antiallergic shots and saved him. Luckily, his family was sensible enough to note down that he was allergic to these drugs. So he is never prescribed them. Be a sensible family member.

It is always useful to have a bracelet around your wrist with details like blood group, allergy, or allergies, or medical conditions like diabetes, heart disease and an emergency contact number in case of an accident or epilepsy.

The Nazis had their blood groups tattooed upon their arms, because they were very systematic about such matters. And this was how many Nazi war criminals were identified later. However, we do not have to take such extreme and painful steps unless we are accident prone and we need blood ever so often.

Accidents Just Waiting to Happen

Many men and women around the house do not normally take care about health precautions, and so accidents happen. And then they say in a very apologetic tone, "I was certain that the child could not reach that medicine. He must have got to it somehow."

That means that if you have a child in the family, make sure that the medicines, drugs, and even washing liquids are out of reach. Many medicines are now being packaged in childproof packages, but they are definitely not foolproof. This reminds me of a Reader's Digest joke. An old lady got a medicine from the chemists, but it was packaged in a childproof bottle. She could not open it, and neither could the chemist! So he just said," all right, Mrs. XYZ, just go outside, and whistle up any kid playing in the street. He is going to open it for you."

Accidental poisoning has a high mortality rate going among little children.

Throw away the drugs, which are not in use or whose potency date has expired.

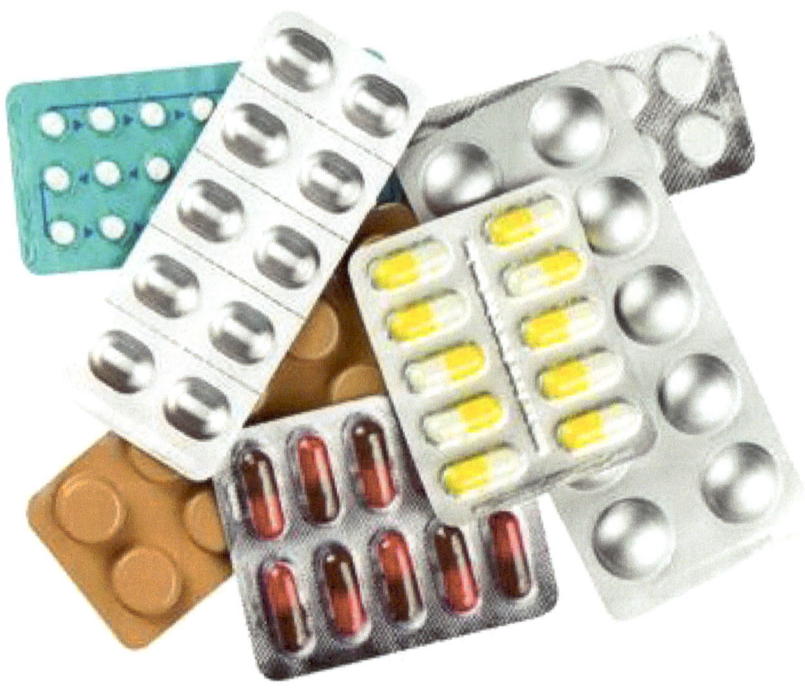

Data expired? Get rid of them in a safe way, by asking your doctor what to do with them. You may give them to him for safe disposal.

Keep a list of emergency telephone numbers – of your doctor, hospital and ambulance, the fire department, and police, stuck to the wall in front of your phone. You may also want to key them in in your cell phone. Teach your children how to press the right buttons in an emergency.

In case of an emergency, nobody has the time to go around searching for emergency telephone numbers, because they are too worried or scared.

Taking Medical Health Training

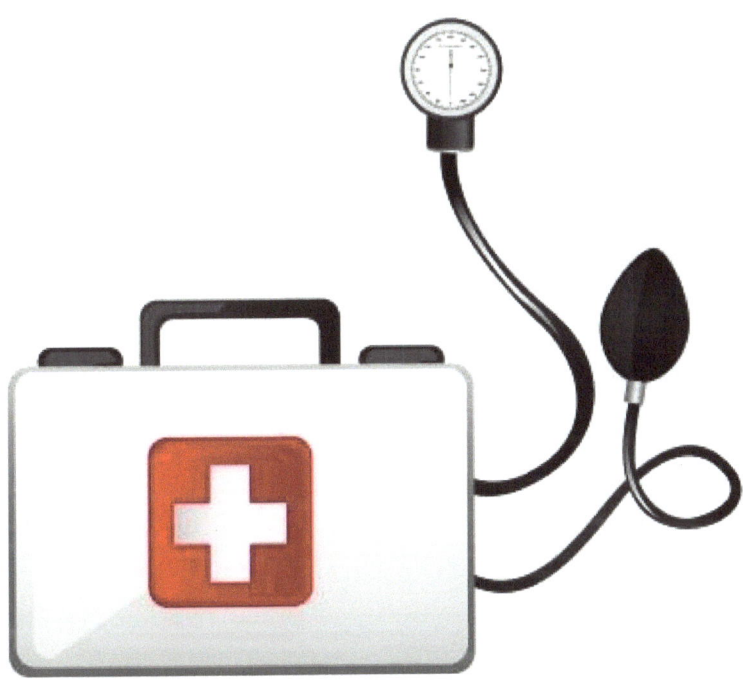

Nowadays, it is always helpful to take some time out, and get some training done in your local Red Cross center. You are going to learn first aid techniques, like how to treat burns, and other emergency treatment measures and procedures, if there is a history of heart disease, in your family.

Many of patient of heart attacks have been saved by emergency heart pumping by a family member, or even mouth to mouth CPR has revived drowning victims. It is better to be prepared than to be sorry, and wake up at two in the morning thinking *if only*.

Attention to the Family's Diet

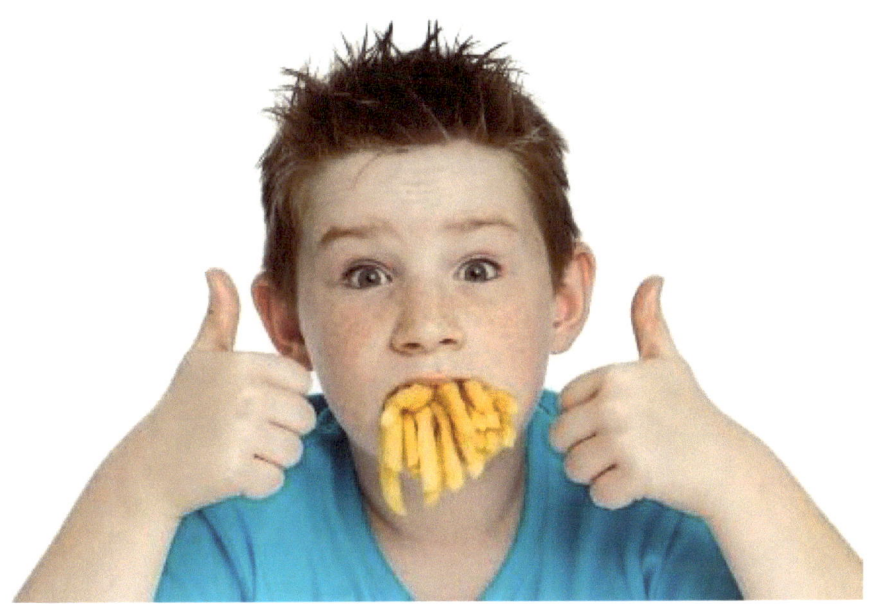

Mom is her kid's worst enemy here because she does not check the things he is eating.

In many parts of the East, obesity is still considered to be the symbol of prosperity. That is because many people have seen very hard times down the ages, and the idea that a person has enough of food, which can make him grow fat has come down as a symbol of a prosperous family.

That is why even today mother stuff their children with all sorts of food, which make them look fat, obese, and bloated and pave the way to future ill health.

All junk foods, and cold drinks are harmful for children and infants. The idea that a fat baby is a healthy child is nonsense, but this idea is very prevalent in the East.

Mother should concentrate upon a well-balanced diet, eggs, milk, fruit juices and healthy snacks instead of popcorn, Coca-Cola, corn syrup based foods, etc., Potato chips should be a definite no-no.

If your children really cannot do without potato chips, I would suggest trying out this recipe.

Cannot Do without Junk Food?

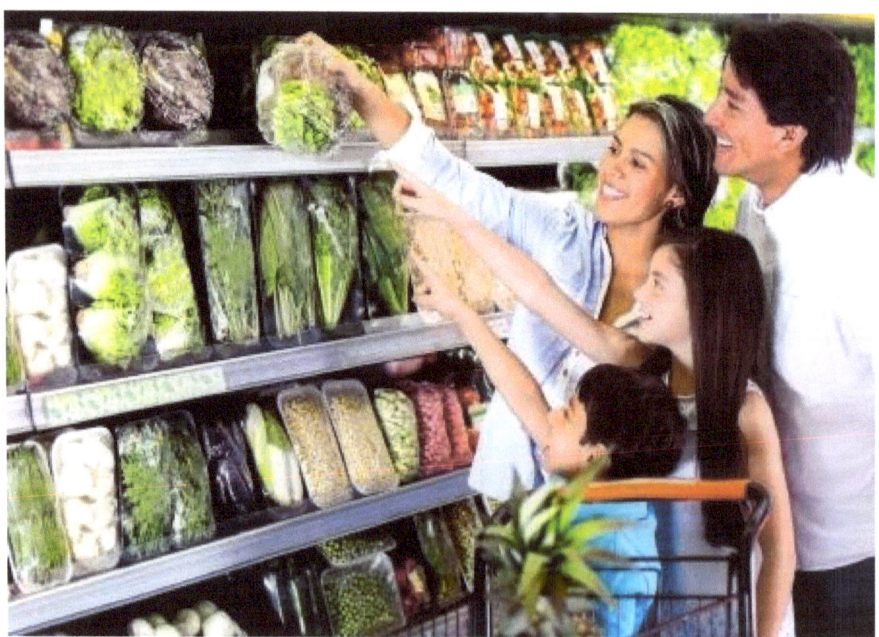

They know what is good for them. But a majority of us still go in for fatty junk food.

Can you believe it that the junk food, which you like to eat so much outside, can be made at home, with hamburgers, tomatoes, green lettuce, onions, cheese, tomato ketchup and anything else you wish. Make sure that the amount of greens are more in your whole-wheat bread sandwiches. Do not add too much salt. When you start eating healthy, you are not going to consider this as junk food, because you are eating natural stuff with nutrients instead of heavily fried foods.

Potato Chips at Home

Put eight large potatoes in ice cold water for half an hour. Grate them very finely on a Chip grater to make paper thin wafers. Fry them on nonstick fry pans, or just use a touch of olive oil. Microwave cooking like you do popcorn can also cook and crisp them. Season with spicy salt and enjoy. Now this is definitely not junk food.

Spicy Salt Healthy Mix – to Sprinkle on Salads

This is a tasty mix, which is normally used as a sprinkle in the East. It is very healthy, because it has spices and other natural ingredients in it. It is also going to have rock salt/black salt in it, which is much better than processed sodium chloride.

Take six spoonfuls of **cumin seed**. Place them on the oil less griddle, and stir continuously on a low heat. This cumin seed is going to change color. It is also going to give out a powerful fragrance as it is roasted. When it turns golden brown in color, remove, allow cooling, and then grind the seeds.

Place immediately in an airtight glass bottle. This roasted cumin seed is going to be used to add spice to all your dishes, with a little bit of salt and pepper. It is an excellent digestive.

Now, collect some **onion, ginger and garlic flakes** – depending on how strong you want their presence in the salt. These flakes are definitely going to lose their power after they have been dried out, when compared to the original.

Onion Flakes

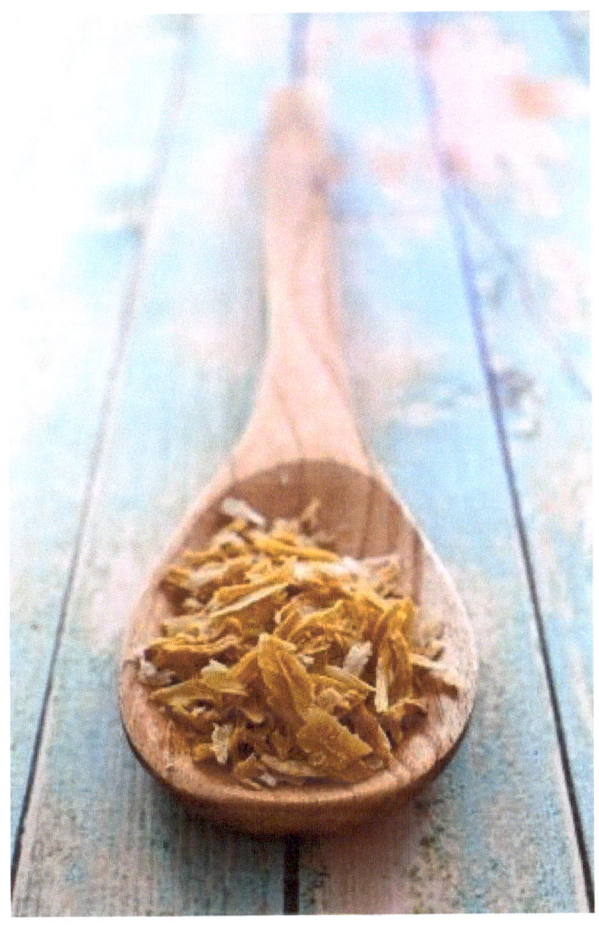

So you can put anywhere between 2 to 3 spoonfuls of each. Onion flakes and ginger flakes can easily be made by slicing them up thin, and then allowing them to dry in the sun, or on the lowest temperature in your oven till all the water has been evaporated. You may also want to use a desiccator/dehydrator.

Now add for teaspoons each of **powdered cinnamon, powdered allspice, powdered cardamoms, coriander seeds, half a teaspoonful of red cayenne pepper, one teaspoonful of black pepper and 2 teaspoons of aniseed** to this mixture. You may want to roast all of them – one at a time, please – if you want a really nice and aromatic mixture. Blend together into a fine powder.

Now take 12 teaspoons of **powdered rock salt** or 8 teaspoons of **powdered black salt**. Add this to this mixture, and blend again. Filter and keep grinding until you have a really fine powder.

This is what I call my allspice healthy spice mixture. Seriously speaking, I cannot do without it, and the amount of this salt, I sprinkle on my food is minimal. So if anybody says that I am eating too much salty food , and that is bad for my liver and kidney, I can just give her the best sneer of my extensive repertoire. I often do that.

You may want to add any more herbs, like dried sage, parsley, dried Oregano, bishops Weed, and thyme to this mixture. I keep trying new combinations of different spices, when I am making up this mixture, but I do love the garlic/onion/ginger combination as a base. And of course rock salt or black salt.

Do not encourage children to eat in between meals. Bad eating habits learned in childhood are going to last throughout their lives and they are going to find it difficult to change their eating habits when they grow up.

Taking Care of Your Patient at Home

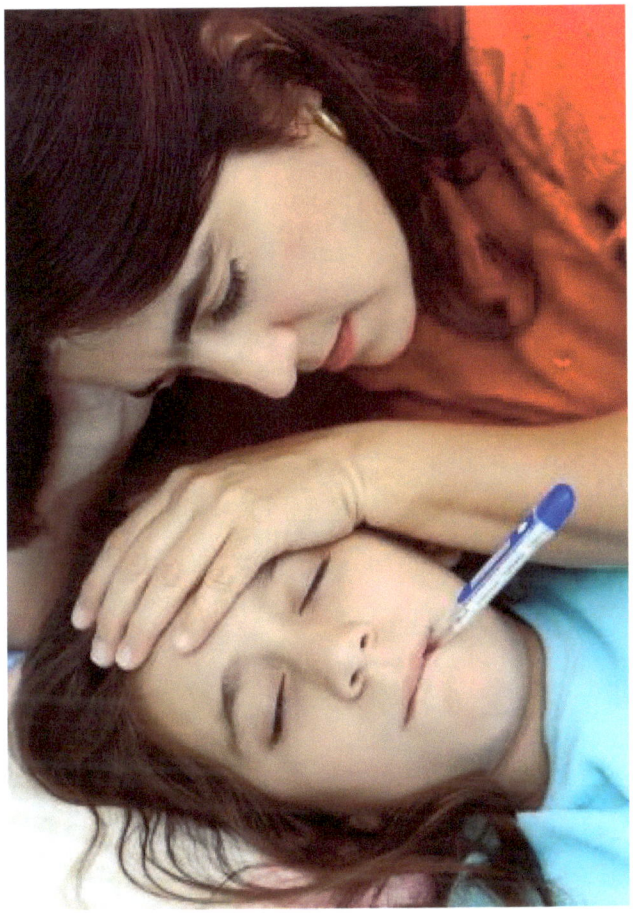

Of course, in this day and age of medical care and achievements, home nursing is a relatively neglected activity. But however, any home maker would be glad to know the finer points of home nursing just in case.

Take for example, the appearance of the winter season bringing with it: colds, influenza and such tiresome ailments which do not necessarily need the patient to be taken to the hospital for a repairing lease.

Coughs and colds get aggravated because people have a tendency to be cooped up in badly ventilated and enclosed areas as to preserve the heat. And thus the infection is spread easily. When it is a cold day, a brisk-paced run or even a swim would help you keep healthy.

However if the cold has managed to catch you it is immediately the responsibility of the lady who runs the house to look after you! How does the lady managed to keep herself fit to keep in good condition to nurse you?

First of all, the nurse has to make sure that the patient is encouraged to go to bed. Because anyone who feels feverish is miserable and in a bad temper, it is the easiest way to get them from under your feet. But on the other hand, if the patient has an infection in the upper breathing passages, lying shall only make him breathe more shallowly and this is not good remedy for such infections.

The semi-flat lying position makes the lungs get congested and thus increases the symptoms. Also lying down makes the infectious matter from the nasal passages to move downwards towards the chest.

Thus the chances of infection are increased.

So the patient must be well wrapped up and settled into a comfortable chair with the foot rest. He can be kept occupied watching TV, listening to music and just relaxing, with his lungs getting enough of oxygen. Make sure he has a hot water bath before he is put into bed. This will make him even more willing to go to sleep!

The best way to get a patient to sleep comfortably as to give them an aspirin and hot milk , along with the doctor's medications. Spread a thin layer of Vaseline and camphor over the patient's upper lip. This will keep the nasal passages cleared. A good thin film of an inhalant Vaporub rubbed upon the chest makes breathing easier.

Medications

We are fortunate that we have plenty of mild antibiotics like aspirin and paracetamol which can be given to relieve headaches, aches and pains and also reduce fever. Paracetamol is normally given to people who have a tendency for stomach upsets.

If there is chest congestion, Vaporubs are best. In the West, a tincture of Benzoin called Friar's Balsam is very widely used, and if you have somebody going to the UK, you would do worse than get a bottle of it.

Cough mixtures are only to be used if there is a dry cough. They can be rectified by a soothing linctus. But if the chest is congested it is necessary for a patient to cough and remove the waste.

A doctor should be involved only when the patient is very old or very young. If the same symptoms persist for longer than a couple of days, then it is absolutely necessary for a doctor to be consulted. Never take any chances with any chest infection going out of control!

Making a Natural VapoRub

Add seven drops of eucalyptus oil and one teaspoonful of powdered camphor to 50 g of petroleum jelly [Vaseline]. Apply this on the chest, massage in circular motions for about 10 minutes and then cover the patient with a warm covering. I also use three drops of mint oil, but that is overkill.

The Patients' Diet

Please be sure that the patient has plenty of fluids at his bedside table. Best is of course lemon juice with salt and sugar /honey.

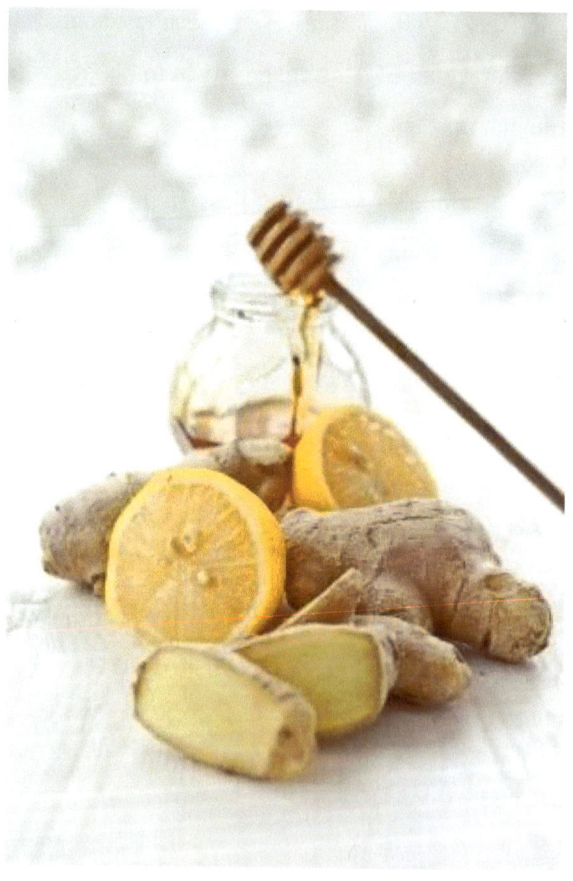

Honey and lemon juice is excellent for invalids

People begin to think that in winter we do not need so many liquids, and thus they get dehydrated. These fluids are absolutely necessary because they flush out all the toxic wastes. For anyone with a chest infection or cold, build up of toxic wastes will prove a setback for recuperation.

If you can dilute orange juice with a mineral water, possibly the patient will think himself compensated during his sickness.

Food for the Sick

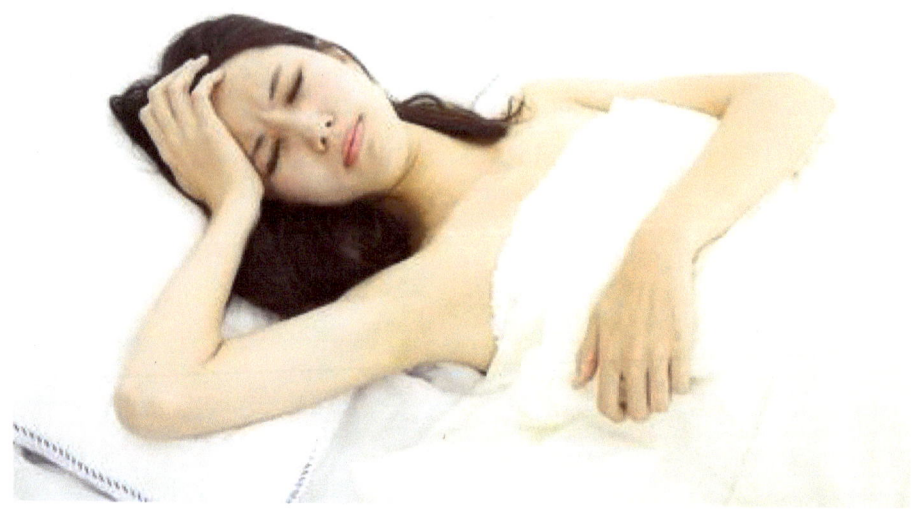

Some people say that a cold has to be fed and the fever has to be starved. This is just an old wife's tale. Healthy, restorative and regular nourishment is necessary for the patient. However children may stop eating during fever, but as long as they have plenty of water and juice to drink, they are all right. They shall immediately gain lost weight, the moment they are restored to health.

The most easily digested foods are Sago pudding(tapioca) and chicken broth.

Recipe for Invalid Chicken Broth

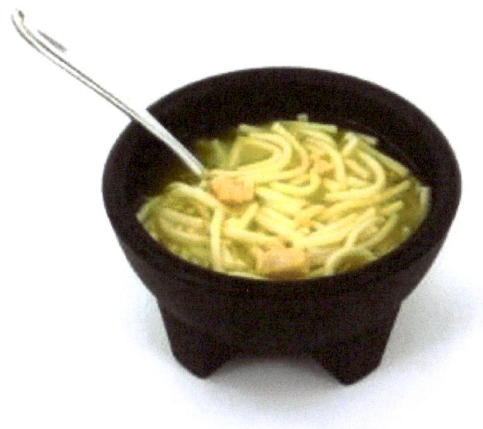

This is chicken soup with noodles

250 grams of chicken pieces, 1 cup milk, six cups water, salt to taste,1/4 cup flour, half cup chopped onions, 1 cup diced potatoes and 1/4 cup barley.

This is the most easily digested and restorative broth ever made.

In a pot, combine the chicken the barley, the milk and water and bring to a boil. Cook slowly until the chicken is tender. Add the potatoes, onions and salt to taste. As soon as you find the broth beginning to thicken, make a paste of the flour in a cup and add it to the mixture. Make sure there are no lumps. You can remove the meat from the pieces, after they are well cooked and tender and put them in the soap bowl.

In fact it is a scientifically proven fact that chicken soup is the best nourishment for colds.

If the patient wants to have something like a stuffed omelette, give him a French or a Spanish one. Otherwise, you can always give him a healthy basic egg omelette, so that he can get the essential nutrients.

Basic Egg Omelets

A stuffed omelet like Spanish omelette is going to be good for your patient when he is recuperating.

3 eggs, salt and pepper, 6 table spoons milk, and 3 tablespoons butter.

Beat the eggs thoroughly in a bowl. Add salt, pepper, and milk. Then place the butter in the frying pan and melt it. Pour in the mixture. Cook it slowly, lifting the edges of the cooking egg towards the center of the frying pan. Keep tipping the pan. Fold half of the omelette, over the other and serve immediately.

For **French omelets**, we use six egg whites, beaten in 6 tbsp. water. In another bowl, we combine the yolks and the salt and pepper, keep beating until the yolks are frothy. Now fold whites in to the yolk mixture. Place the butter in a frying pan and melt it. Let it cook slowly over low heat for one minute until the bottom of the omelette is slightly browned.

Place the frying pan under a grill until the top is slightly brown. Fold it in to half and serve immediately.

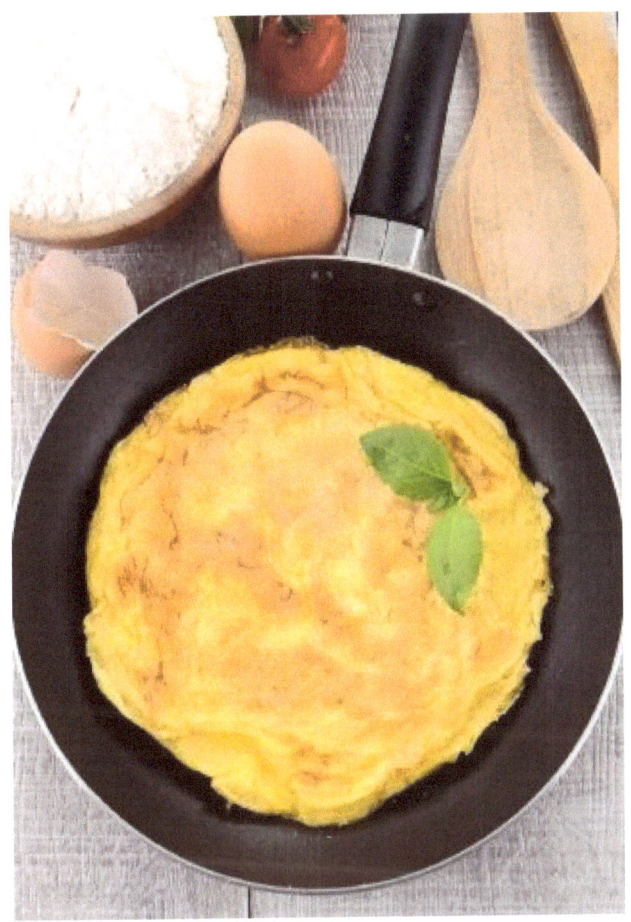

The **Spanish omelette** is normally given when the person feels like having a hearty meal.

You need five double spoons of oil, three fourths cup chopped onions, half cups chopped green peppers, 3 tomatoes in A paste, salt pepper and chilies to taste, four eggs and half a cup of milk.

In a frying pan cook the onions and the green peppers in the oil. Then add the tomato paste, water, salt and chilies. Cover and bring to a boil. Lower the heat and uncover.

Cook this mixture for eight or 10 minutes. In the bowl, combine the eggs, milk salt and pepper. In another frying pan, heat some more oil, add the egg mixture and cook it. Lift up the omelette as it sets. Keep tilting the edges until the egg is cooked. Serve it with sauce.

Traditional Lemon Squash (Nimbu pani- lit- lemon water)

8 tsp of sugar, 6 tbsp squeezed lime juice, 4 cups of water, salt to taste , crushed ice to serve. Mix them all together and place them in the fridge. Keep drinking as often as possible, especially in the summer or whenever you want to replenish your vitamins C, energy and water level. When you were kids, we managed about four-- 5 glasses of nimbu pani a day and never ever caught a cold in the winters or a sunstroke in the summers.

This nimbupani was also a blessing during the rare occasions when we caught a fever, because warm nimbu pani with lots of salt and pepper four times a day brought us bouncing back and in fighting trim within the week.

Tapioca Pudding

Cooking tapioca pudding for the invalid.
1/3 cups tapioca, soaked in water for 20 minutes.
3 cups of whole milk.
Sugar to taste.

When you are cooking for an invalid, you do not add milky cream, nuts of your choice like raisins and almonds, cardamoms and other spices. That is normally done when this pudding is made for festive occasions in the East. But as we are cooking ordinary healthy food for a patient, we going to keep it basic.

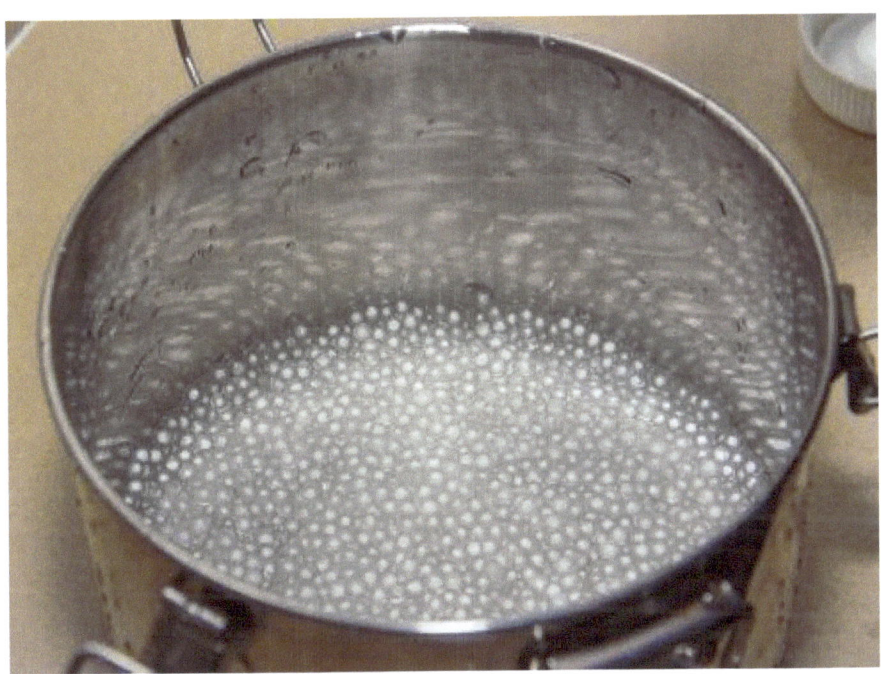

Tapioca pudding is going to solidify and thicken, if you refrigerate it overnight. So the next time you use it, you can add some more milk and heat up again.

Melt the oil in the cooking pan. Put the milk onto boil, on low heat. Now add the now, drained tapioca and keep cooking, stirring continuously. The properly cooked tapioca is going to get translucent within 20 – 25 minutes. Let cool for some time and add sugar before feeding to the invalid.

If you are just heating this as dessert, I would suggest that you fry the dry fruit first in unsalted clarified butter. This is so that the aroma is fixed. These dry fruit along with cardamoms are added after the tapioca is cooked, and before it is frozen.

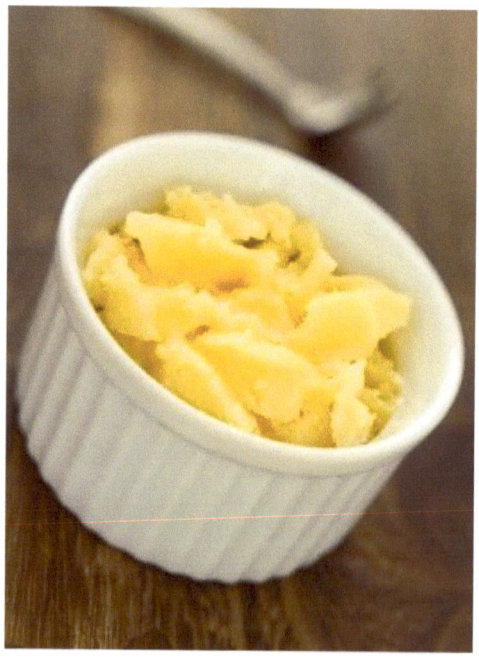

This unclassified butter is called Desi ghee. You do not give it to your invalid, but you do give it to him, while he is recuperating so that he can get healthy again.

Onion Soup

This is what can be given when the patient is recuperating.

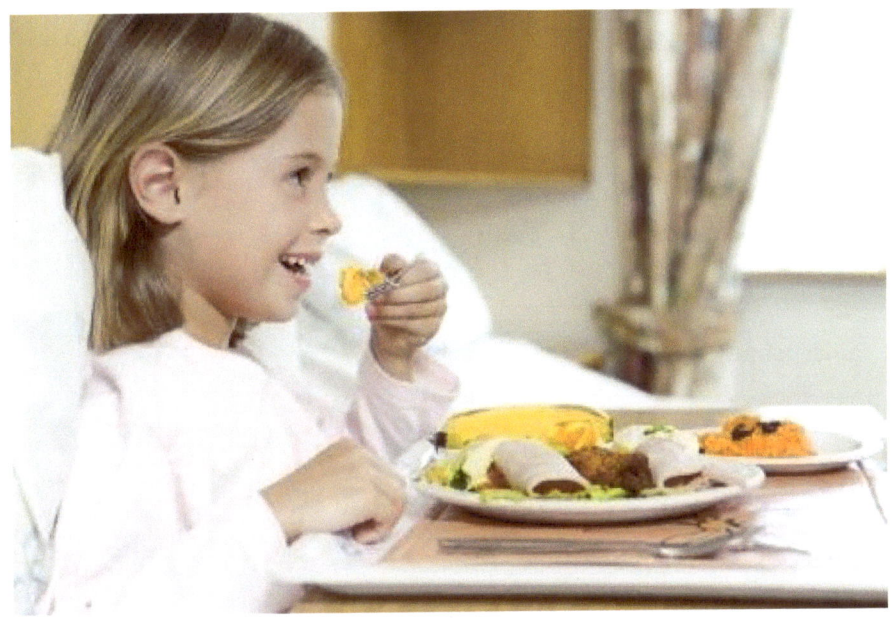

Healthy nutritious food is a must for recuperating patients.

Six onions, finely cut.

4 tablespoons full of butter.

Four cubes of bouillon dissolved in a cup of boiling water.

Three glasses of boiling water.

1 tablespoon full of salt.

1/8 teaspoon celery salt – salt mixed with powdered celery leaves.

1/8 teaspoon Oregano/cilantro

¼ teaspoon parsley leaves

Pinch of pepper

Fry the onions in the butter on low heat so that you do not brown them. When they are nice and soft, put them in the water and add all the other ingredients. Simmer them for 45 minutes, but do not boil this soup too hard. Because this soup must be aged to perfection, put it in the refrigerator for 24 hours before serving. If there is any left, put it back. Reheat it as many times as you wish, and it is going to be tastier every time.

Traditional Tomato Cheese Rarebit

1 tablespoon full of flour.

Half a can of tomato soup – Cambells is best.

¼ teaspoon salt

1 tablespoon Worcestershire sauce

Half a cup of cheese, grated

2 cups of milk.

Add the Worcestershire sauce, and the salt to the tomato soup and then blend the flour in. Cook this in a double boiler by putting the soup container in another container with water. Add grated cheese and heat under a grill until the cheese begins to melt. Add milk slowly and heat it to serving temperature. Now serve this piping hot over hot buttered toast.

To make sure that the water does not go dry, put the jar lid of a can on the bottom of the outdoor boiler. The moment the water gets low, the jar lid is going to rattle.

How to Become a Home Health Aide

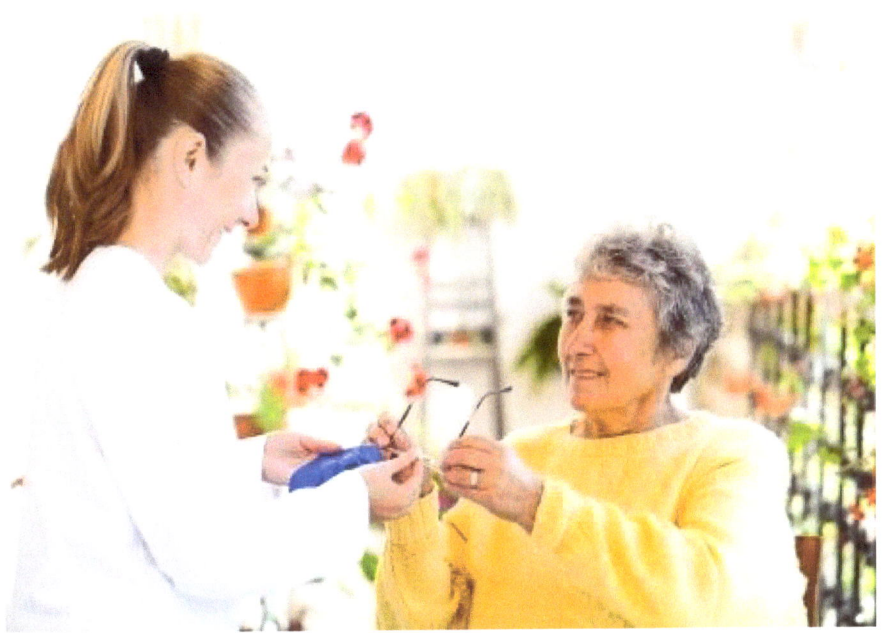

With the demand for experienced and well qualified home health aides in the healthcare sector increasing every year, it is possible that you are looking for tips how to become a home health aide. Well, you have finally chosen a career, which can only be undertaken by a person who is willing and dedicated enough to take care of elderly, sick and disabled patients in their homes.

Many people who cannot provide their loved ones with such professional and caring attention normally hire responsible and trained home health aides to do this work for them. So if you intend to become a home caregiver, here are the points which you need to fulfill –

You have to be more than 18 years of age.

Students enrolling themselves in certified nursing aide CN classes in responsible institutes are going to go through medical checks. They are also going to be tested for substance abuse and a criminal background check is also going to be done on them.

A High School Diploma is desirable, because you will have already studied about the basic topics that you are going to learn in depth, like hygiene, nutrition, biology, physiology and anatomy. These are health related topics which are going to be taught to you in your home health aide classes.

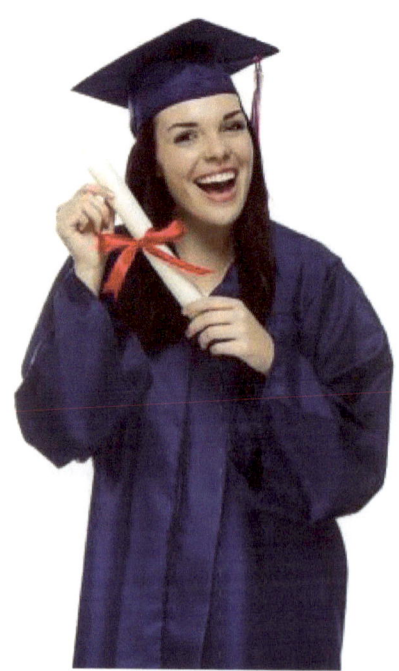

It is necessary that you have proper state approved training given to you through technical or vocational, community colleges, government run institutions, institutions like the Red Cross, and even agencies giving you home healthcare training facilities. After your training has been done, you will need to take the CNA certification exam which is going to be oral, written, and a practical clinical skills test.

Good home health aide training programs are going to be for 75 hours, with 15 hours or more of practical on –hands- skills training in a ward of a hospital or nursing home. These classes are going to be taken by therapists, experienced and registered nurses and also vocational and licensed nurses (LPNs/LVNs). They are going to train you in all the different duties which you are going to undertake as a home health aide, on a regular daily basis.

State Requirements for Home Health Aides

There are different state requirements for home health aides, in different states, so you will need to check them out carefully, before you enroll for home health aide training programs and classes. Some of these states require that you be licensed before you can pick up in her senior job. If your employer has Medicare insurance and reimbursement, you may need to undergo experience and competency tests and evaluation after you have completed your professional training course and program.

This means that you are capable of taking care of all the necessary duties, like grooming and bathing the patient, checking his vital signs and noting it, giving the necessary recommended medication to the patient and other activities which are a part of home health aides' duties. You may be also required to take care of the washing and the sanitization of your patient's clothing and bedding. Remember that this duty does not extend to your taking care of the patient's family's washing and cleaning household chores. You will need to make this clear, at the very onset, before you take up a home health aide job in a private home.

Many people are looking for home healthcare jobs, because that gives them an opportunity to earn anywhere between USD 18,000 to USD 26,000, depending on their experience and knowledge. So even though you may consider this job to be limited in its scope for promotion, you can always save money and train for higher qualifications like registered nurses, orthopedic nurses, geriatric nurses, therapists and psychiatric nurses. The scope is endless, as long as you have the will to undertake such a responsible and conscientious job.

So now that you know how to become a home health aide, look for the CNA training classes available to you in your state or in your city, right now. Some schools are also offering you online training classes, which may suit you if you already have a full-time job.

Conclusion

Did you know that in medieval times, a mother who had all her children surviving because she took good care of them, and make sure that they never fell sick or succumbed to seasonal ailments or epidemics was considered to be a witch and surely in league with the devil. Thank God, we do not live in such superstitious, illiterate and parlous times. Mothers have more sense today, so they know everything about health, nursing, and proper care of their babies and children.

So now that you have learned more about home nursing, and how to take care of an invalid, you may want to use the tips and techniques given in this book. You never know when somebody is going to fall sick at home. You may also have some person in the family who is chronically prone to illnesses. At that time, you find your life revolving around him or her. You want to make sure that he is given the best care, and that can only be done by somebody who really cares for him. So it could either be you or it could be a nursing aide who is qualified and experienced.

Remember that home nursing can be done by anybody who has a little bit of common sense, patience and the ability to take care of a fractious and sick patient. People say that children make the worst patients. That is not so. They are so absolutely patient and thankful that there is somebody to take care of them, that they are as good as gold.

However, they turn out to be bad patients, when they are recuperating, and want to get out of bed like right now. That is when hassled moms and pops begin to wonder what to do with such children, who have bounced back so wonderfully noisily and energetically. Amid bouts of thankfulness that their children are fine now.

Also, I have noticed the same thing in old people. They appreciate the touch of care so much. But unfortunately, many times they do not bounce back because they are too weak. And so we lose them to our great regret.

Do not let that happen to any member of your family, whether child or adult. Good luck go with you and your family.

Author Bio

Dueep Jyot Singh is a Management and IT Professional who managed to gather Postgraduate qualifications in Management and English and Degrees in Science, French and Education while pursuing different enjoyable career options like being an hospital administrator, IT,SEO and HRD Database Manager/ trainer, movie scriptwriter, theatre artiste and public speaker, lecturer in French, Marketing and Advertising, ex-Editor of Hearts On Fire (now known as Solsctice) Books Missouri USA, advice columnist and cartoonist, publisher and Aviation School trainer, ex- moderator on Medico.in, banker, student councilor ,travelogue writer … among other things! One fine morning, she decided that she had enough of killing herself by Degrees and went back to her first love -- writing. It's more enjoyable! She already has 48 published academic and 14 fiction- in- different- genre books under her belt.

When she is not designing websites or making Graphic design illustrations for clients , she is browsing through old bookshops hunting for treasures, of which she has an enviable collection – including R.L. Stevenson, O.Henry, Dornford Yates, Maurice Walsh, C.N.Williamson, Sapper, Bartimeus and the crown of her collection- Dickens "The Old Curiosity Shop," and so on… Just call her "Renaissance Woman" - collecting herbal remedies, acting like Universal Helping Hand/Agony Aunt, or escaping to her dear mountains for a bit of exploring, collecting herbs and plants, and trekking.

Check out some of the other Health Learning Series books at Amazon.com

Health Learning Series on Amazon

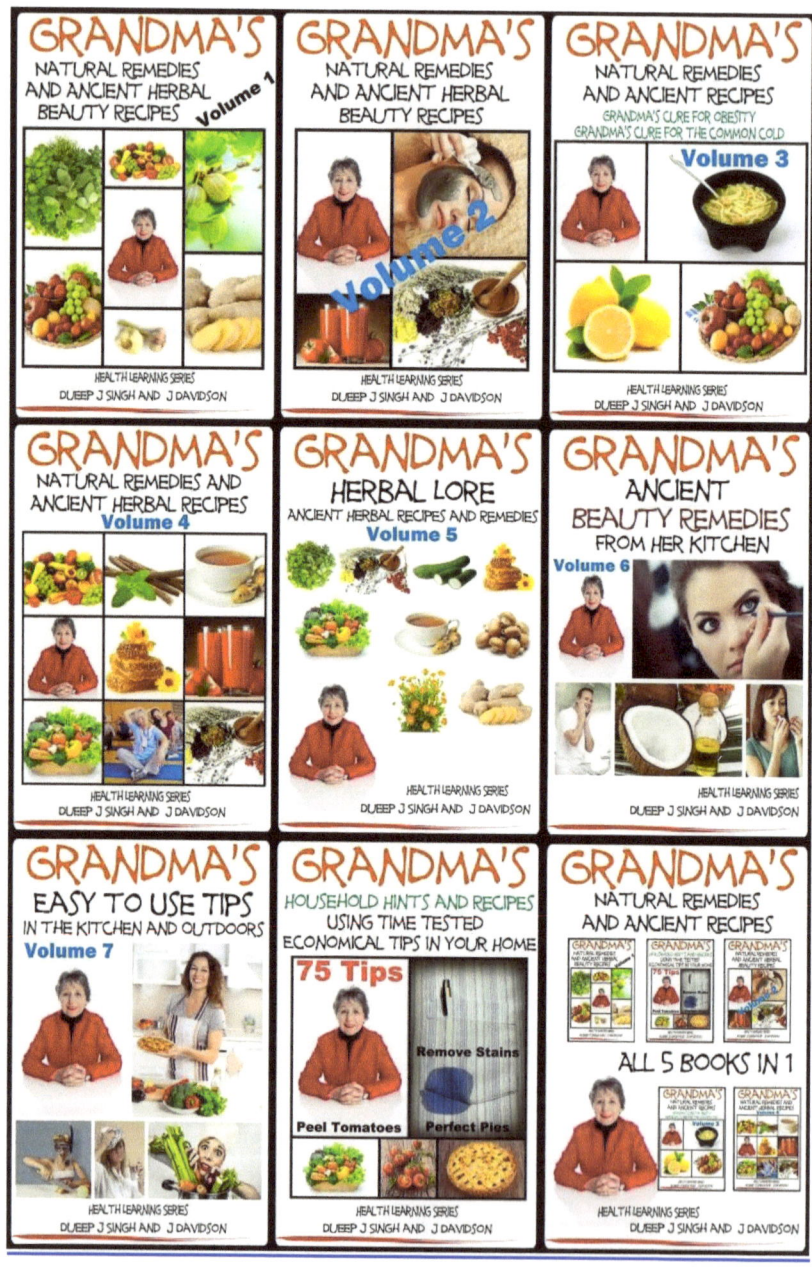

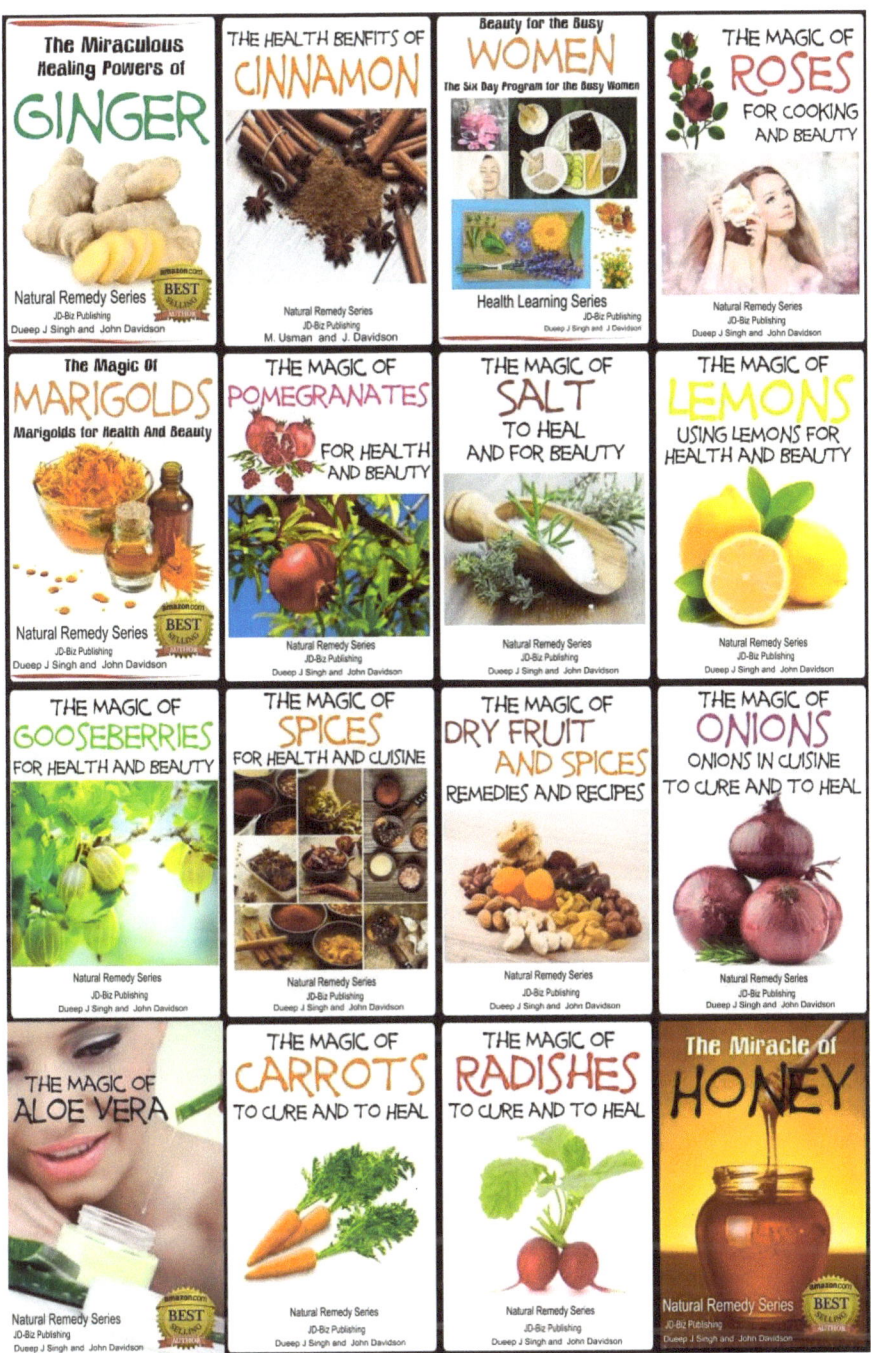

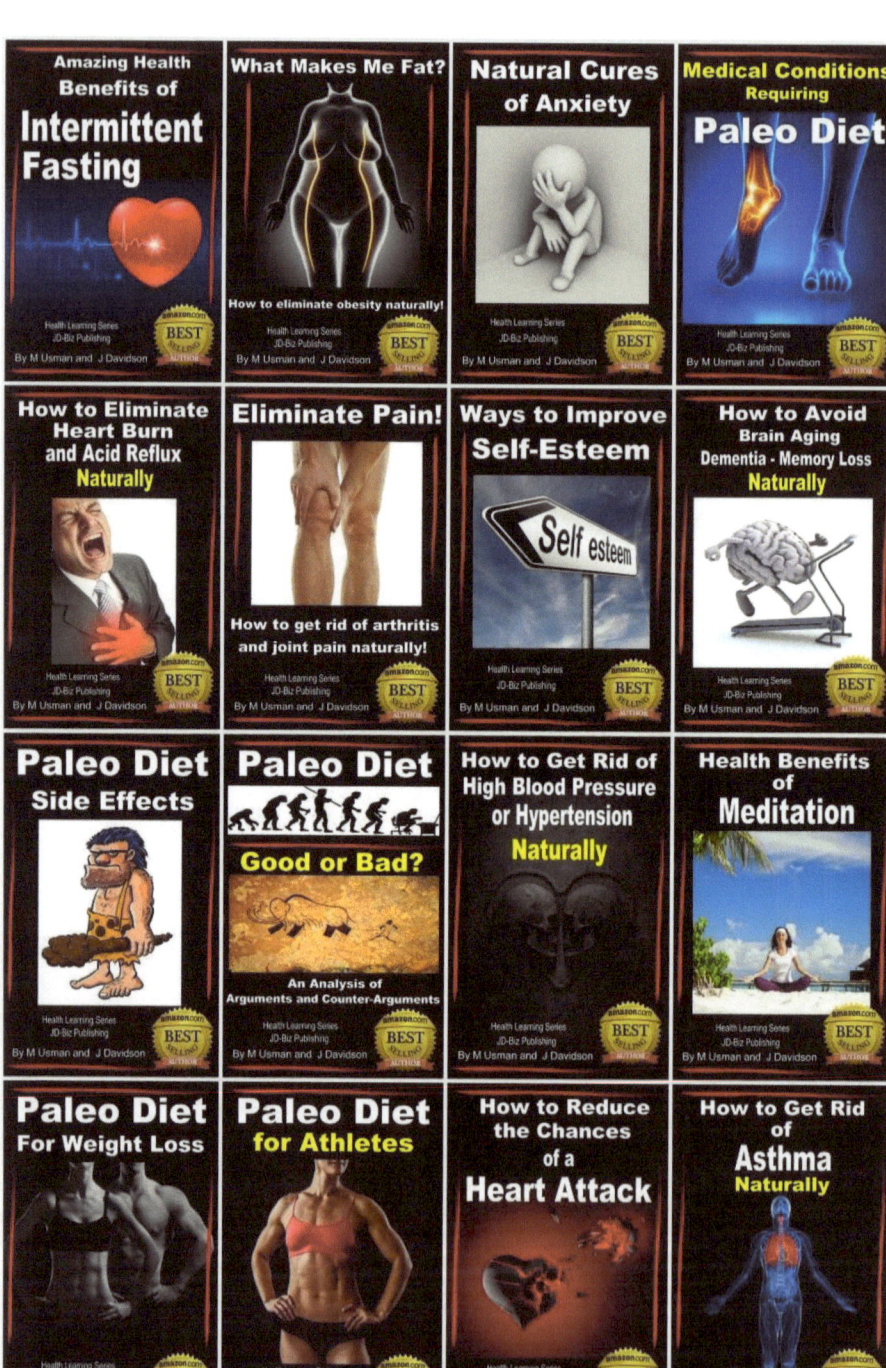

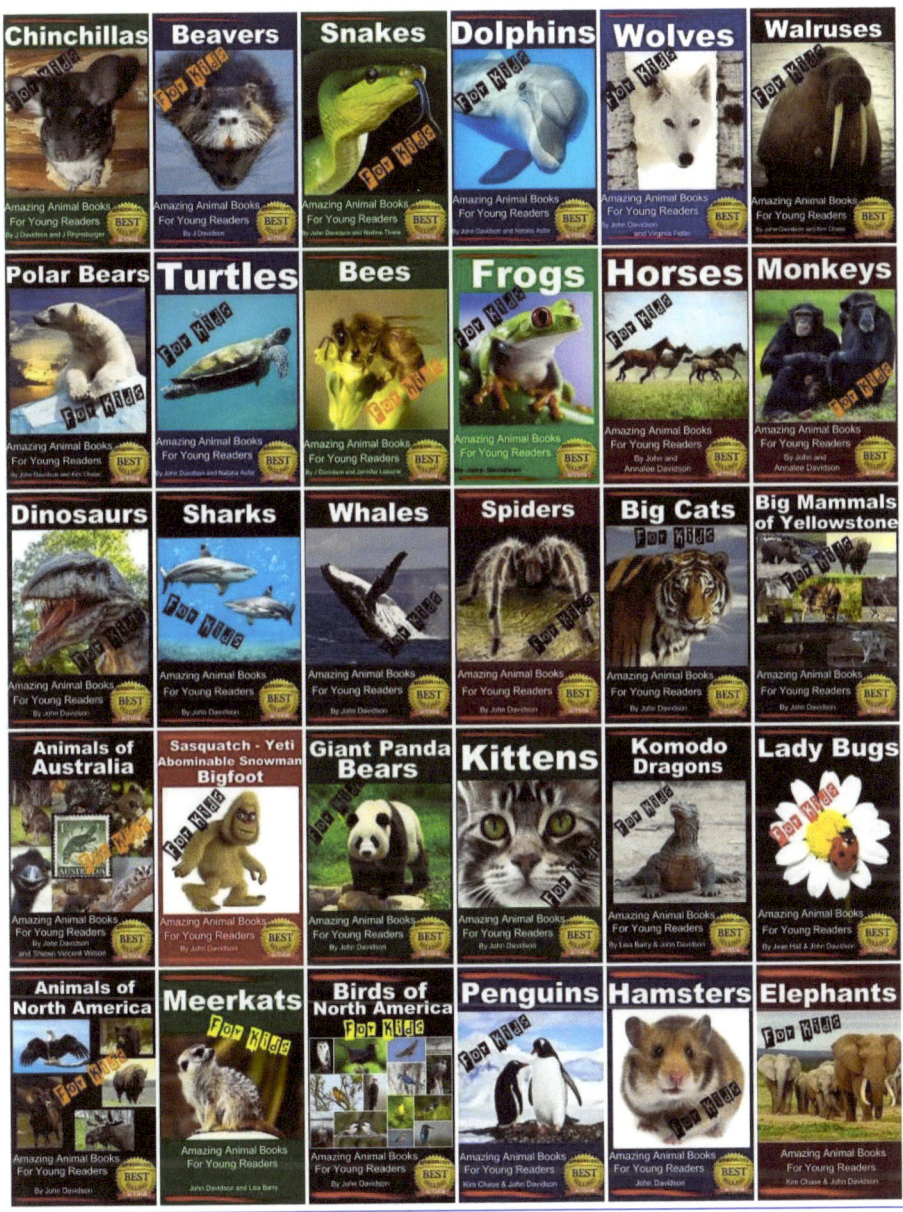

Learn To Draw Series

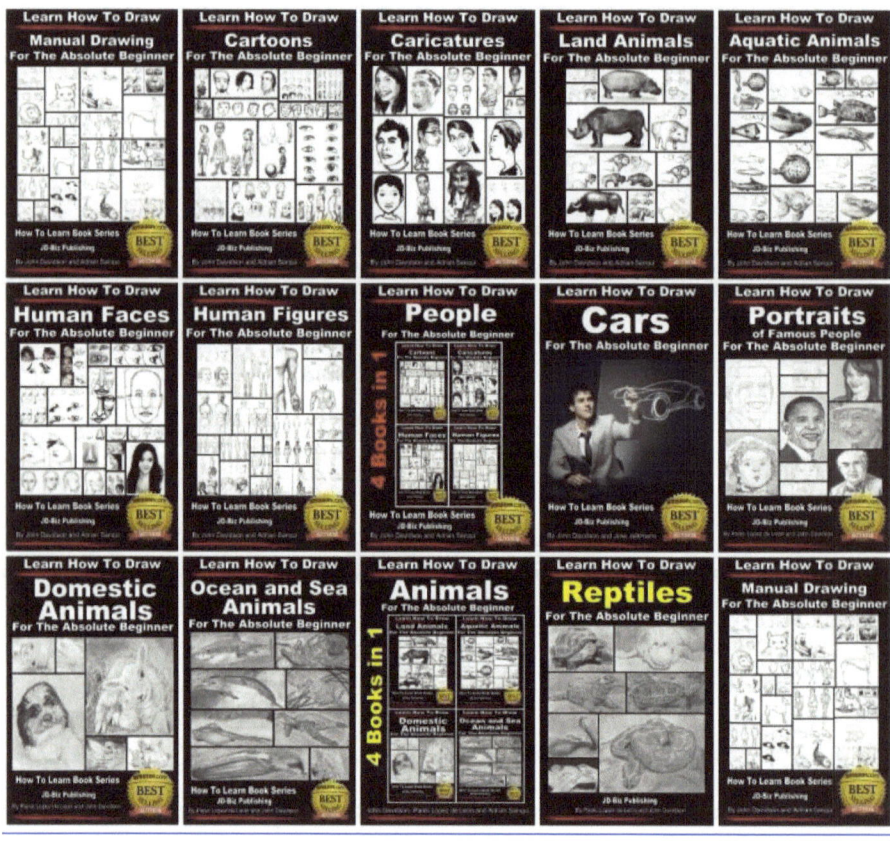

How to Build and Plan Books

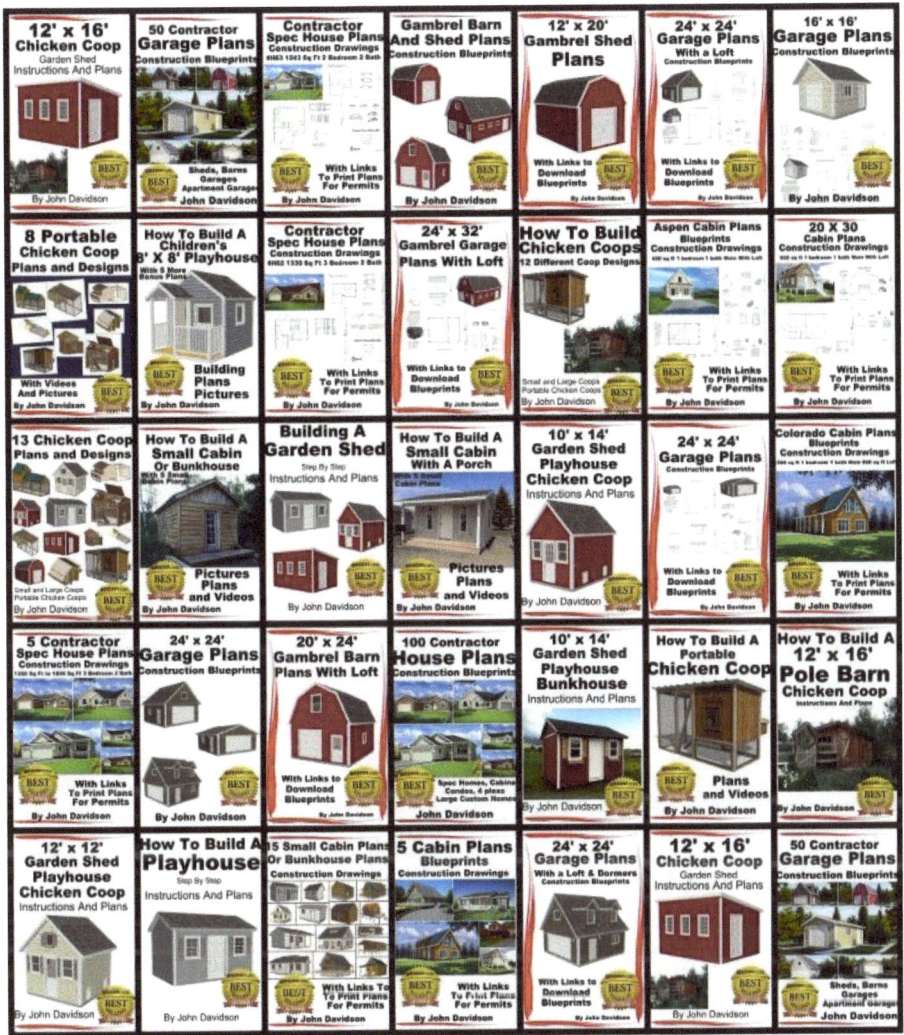

Our books are available at

1. Amazon.com

2. Barnes and Noble

3. Itunes

4. Kobo

5. Smashwords

6. Google Play Books

Download Free Books!

http://MendonCottageBooks.com

Publisher

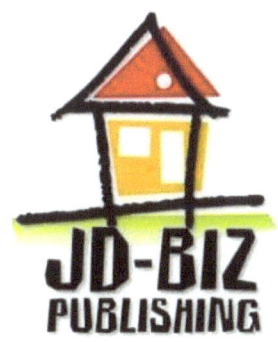

JD-Biz Corp

P O Box 374

Mendon, Utah 84325

http://www.jd-biz.com/

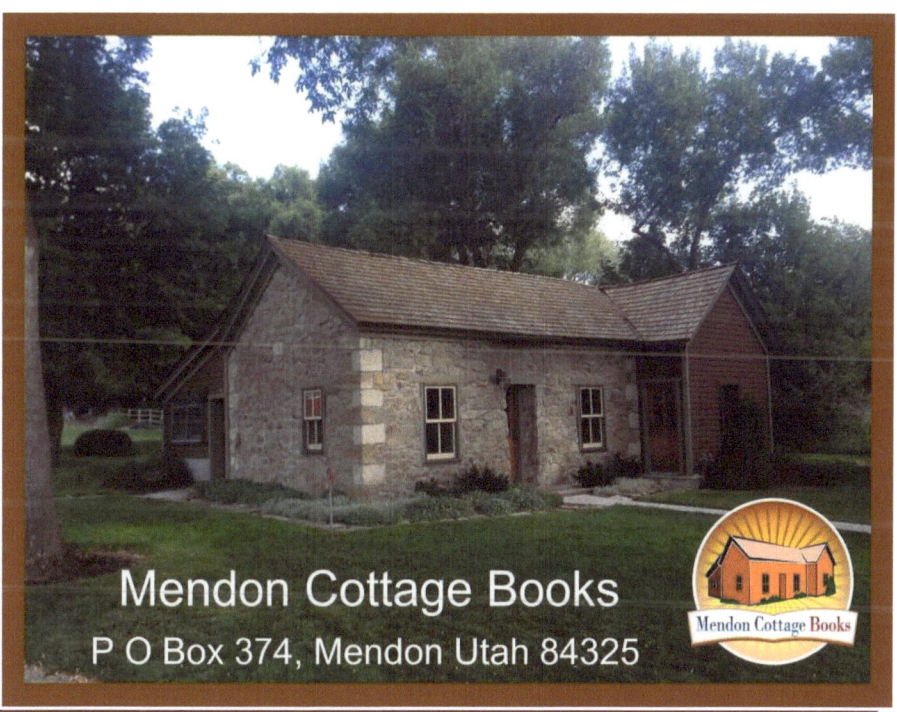

Mendon Cottage Books

P O Box 374, Mendon Utah 84325

www.ingramcontent.com/pod-product-compliance
Lightning Source LLC
Chambersburg PA
CBHW040837180526
45159CB00001B/219